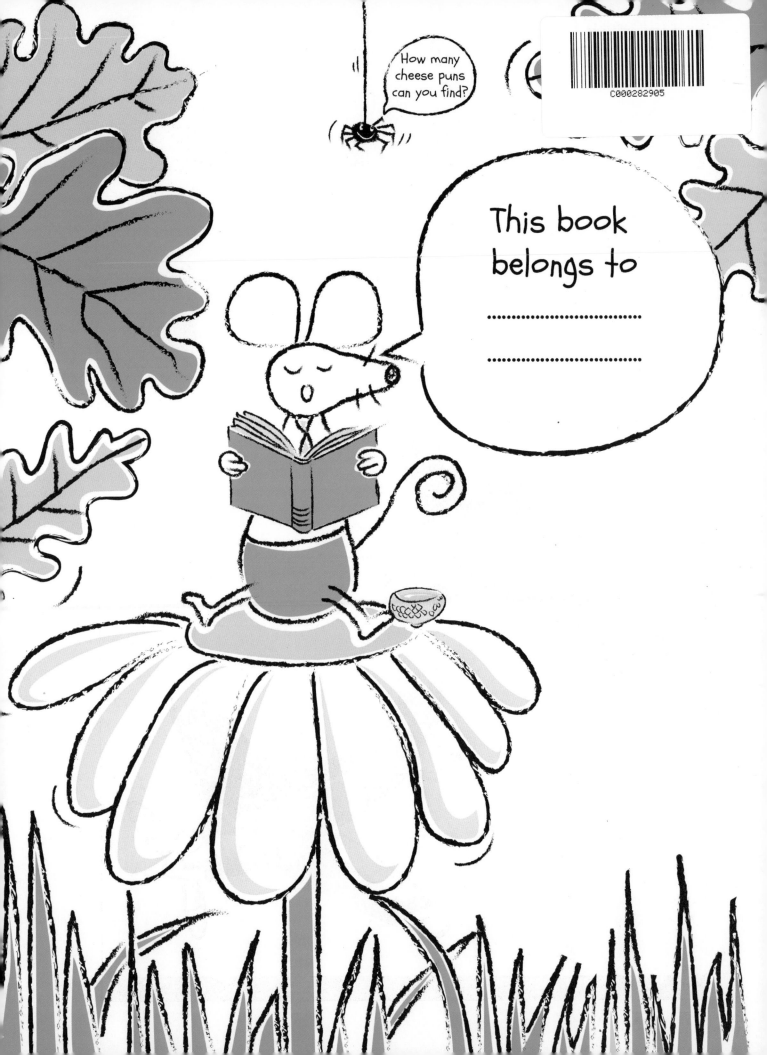

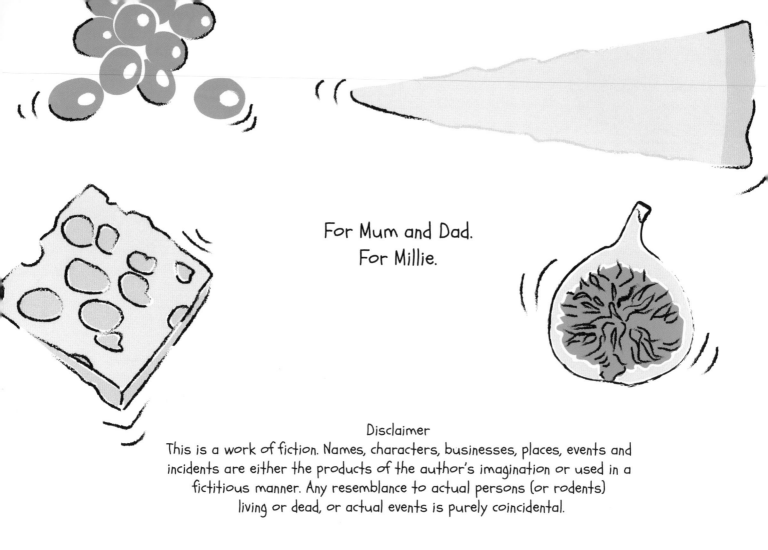

For Mum and Dad.
For Millie.

Disclaimer
This is a work of fiction. Names, characters, businesses, places, events and
incidents are either the products of the author's imagination or used in a
fictitious manner. Any resemblance to actual persons (or rodents)
living or dead, or actual events is purely coincidental.

Paperback: 978-1-7399893-0-9
E-book: 978-1-7399893-1-6
Text and illustration by Cathy Kingham
Edited by Graham Bostock
Artwork support by Bacroom Design

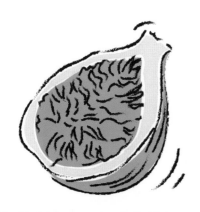
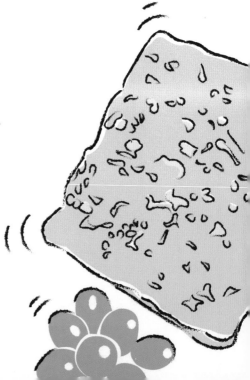

Hector

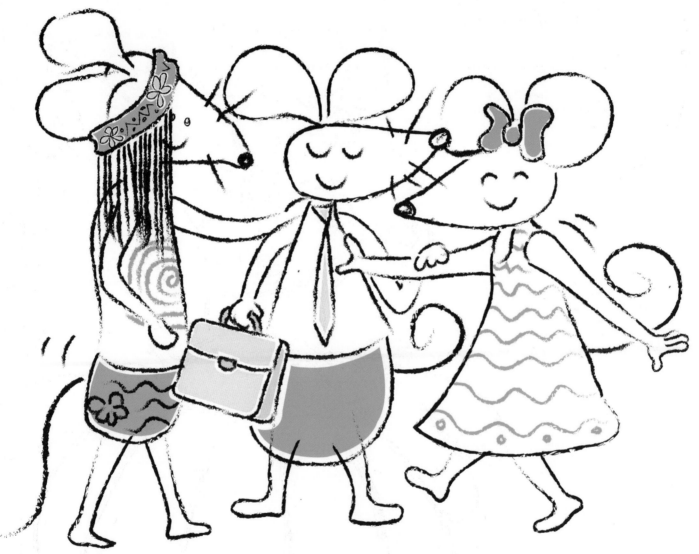

(He works for the public sector)

Written and illustrated by
Cathy Kingham

VERMIN CITY COUNCIL

The New Cheese Distribution Team
(plus an owl, a doctor and a spider)

Hector
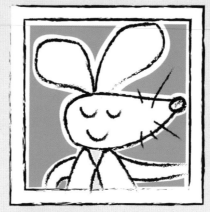
"Hi, I'm Hector and I'm really positive about this exciting new challenge."

Sophia
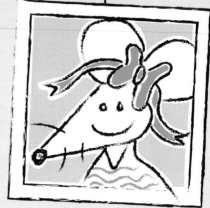
"I'm excited to be joining this new team and meeting my colleagues."

Alfie
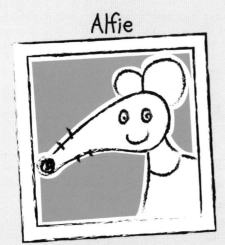
"Cheese and a new challenge! What's not to like?"

Bal
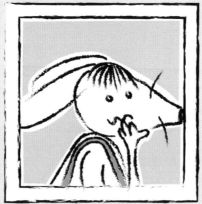
"I really hope I get a nice manager with lots of experience, to support and guide me."

Azure
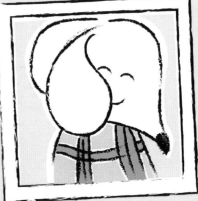
"I've just graduated and I really want to help rodents less fortunate than myself."

Hebe
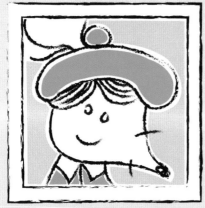
"I'm a really hard worker and always get the job done. A work-life balance is really important to me."

Jackson
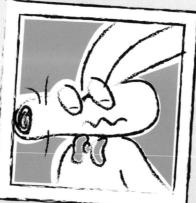
"I have a lot of experience and can't wait to share my ideas with the team."

Finn
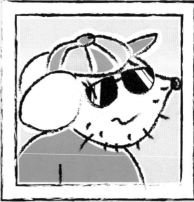
"Wow, working with cheese! That roqueforts my world!"

Benita

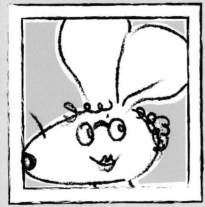

"As a mature rodent, I have a lot of life skills. I have a big family to support."

Dirty Dave

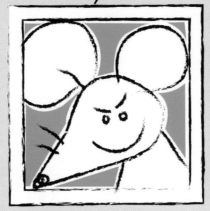

"My aim is to benefit personally, professionally, and financially."

Petrichor

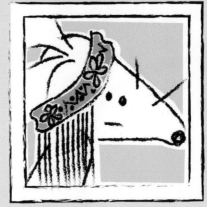

"I love working in the great outdoors, man."

Orion

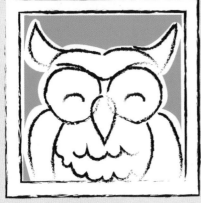

"Life's a hoot!"

Dr Singh

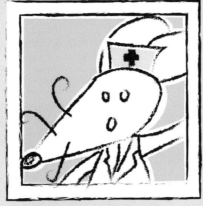

"It's been a tough year at Rodent General."

Hoang

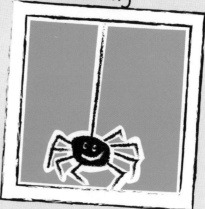

"I see myself as a kind of arachnid advocate. I'm also into web design."

Line Cheese

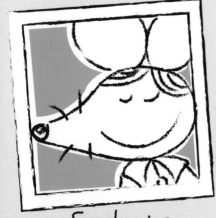

Saccharine

"As a line manager, it is lovely to see fresh, new ~~cannon-fodder~~ talent!"

Team Cheese

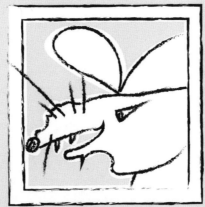

Bernard

"As a team manager, I am committed to the wellbeing and personal development of all staff members."

BIG CHEESE

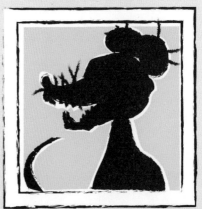

"Together whey will continue to make Vermin City Council great!"

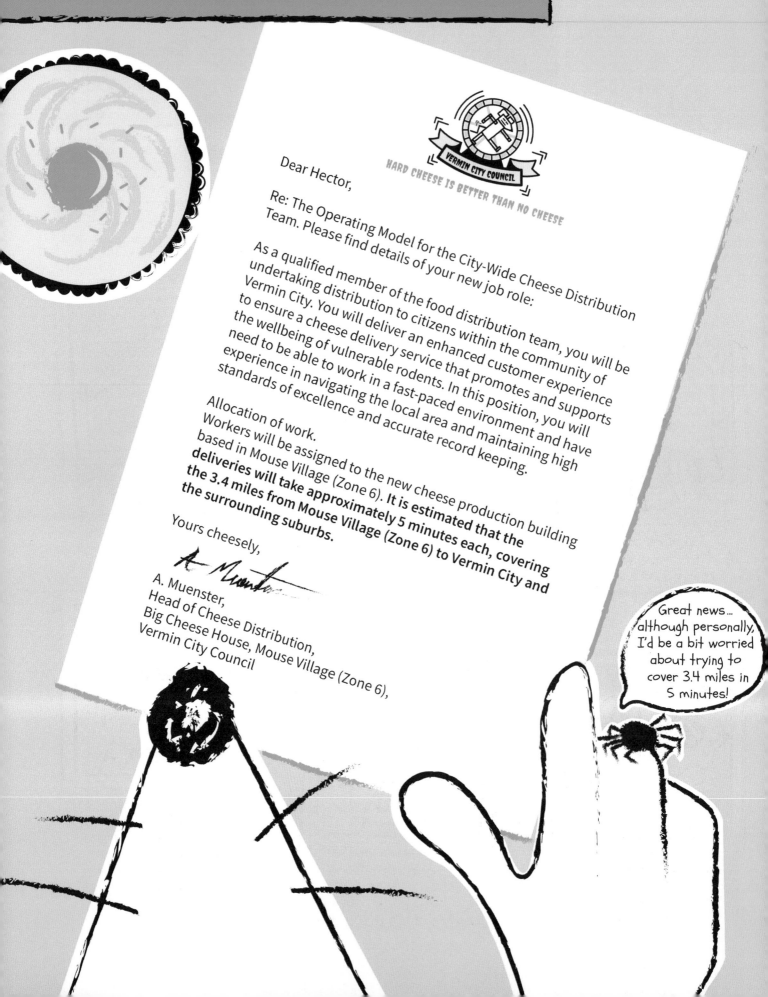

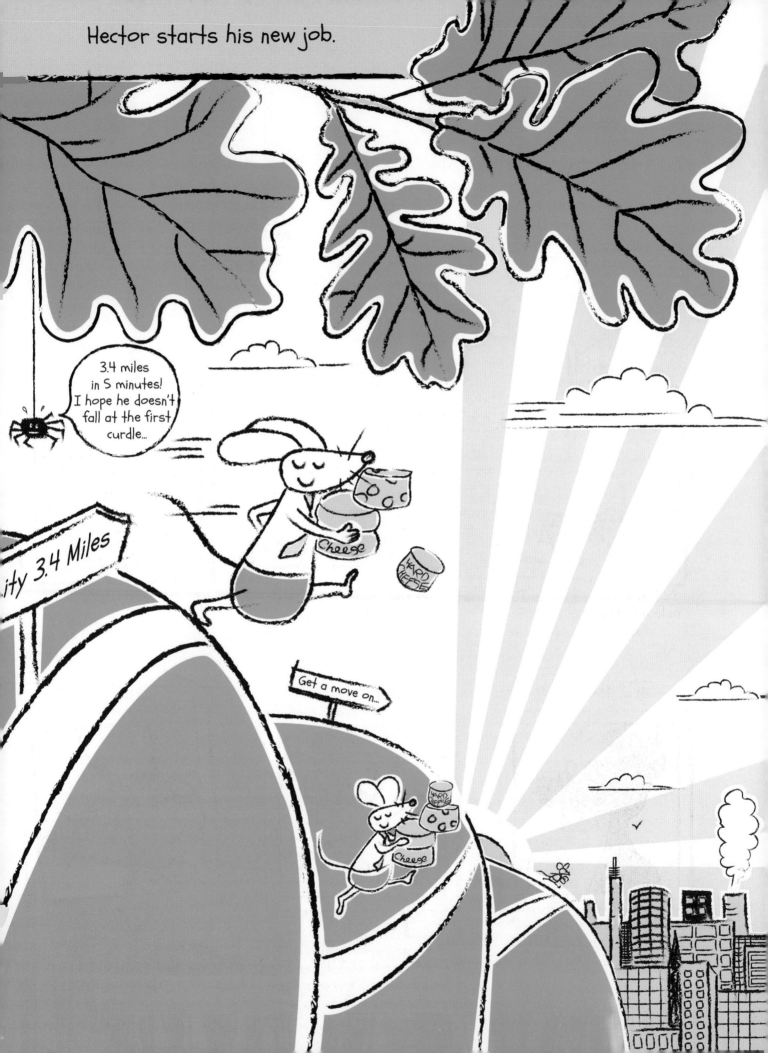

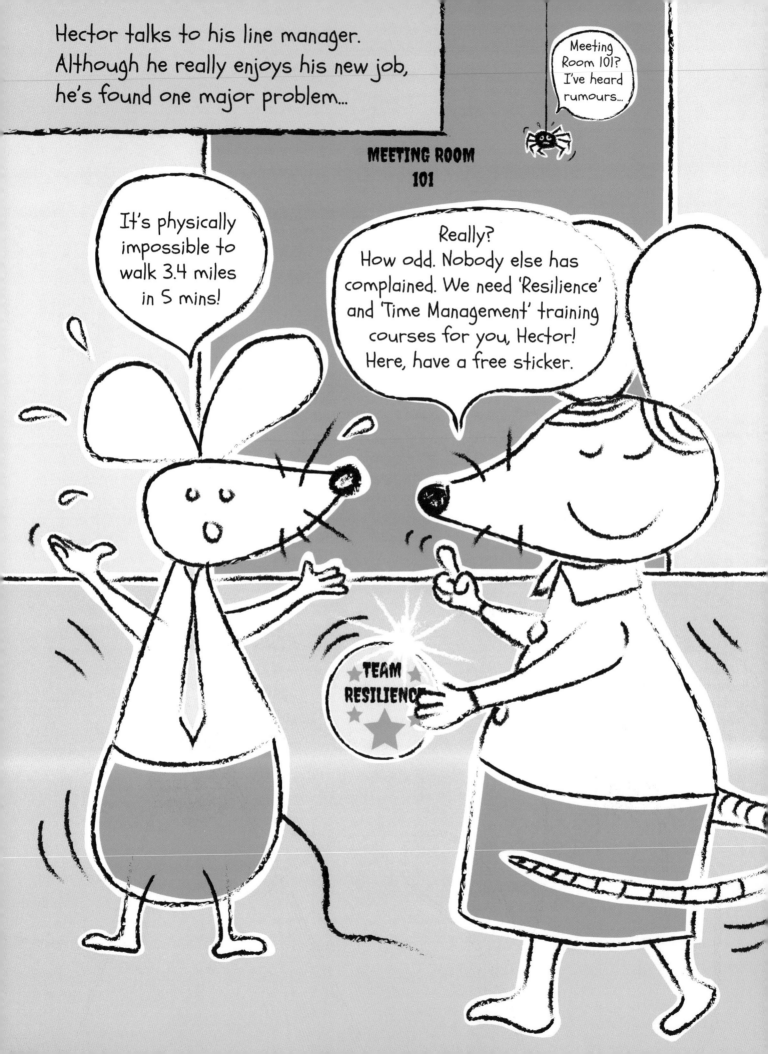

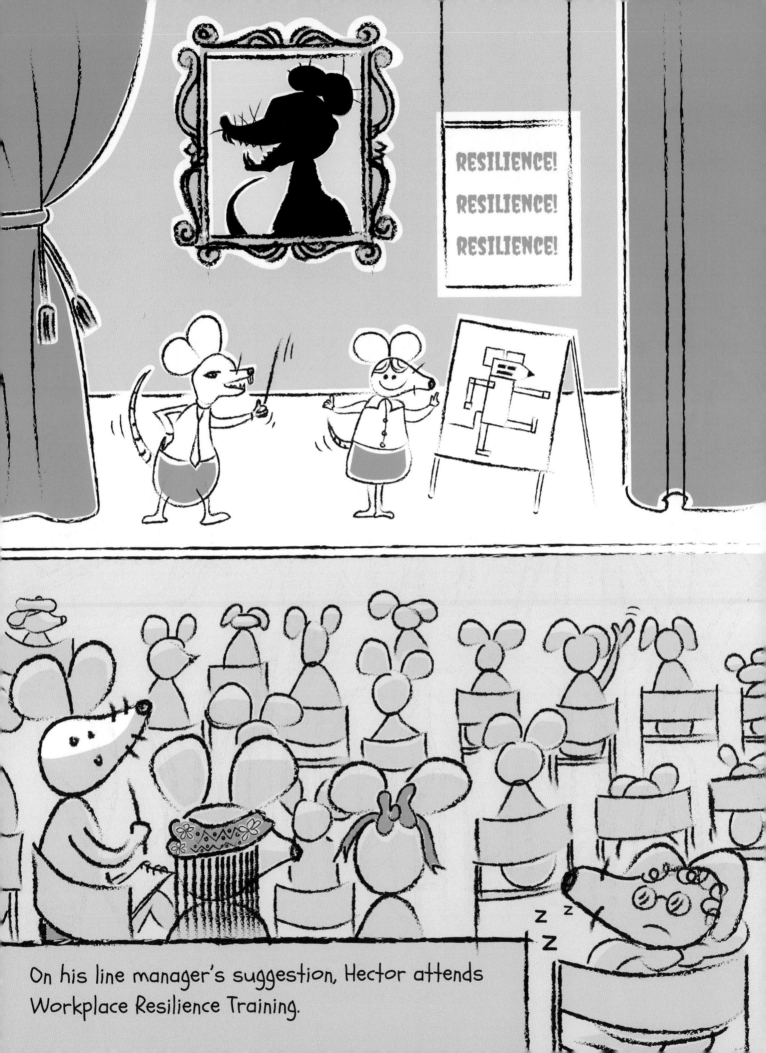

On his line manager's suggestion, Hector attends Workplace Resilience Training.

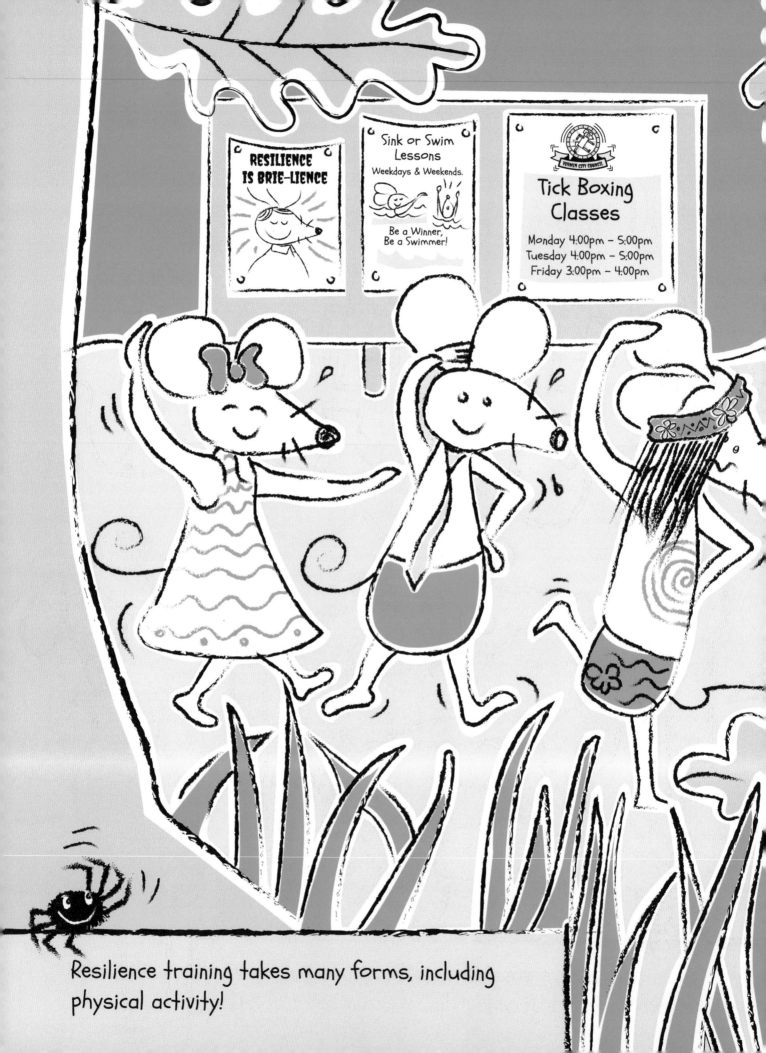

Resilience training takes many forms, including physical activity!

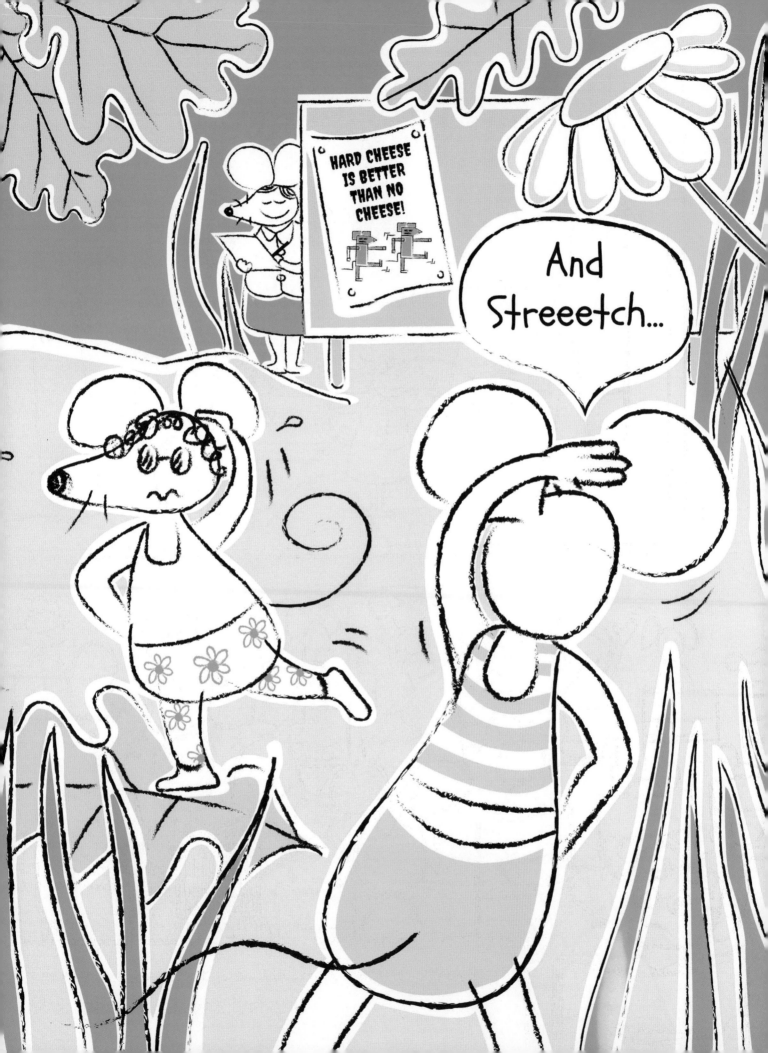

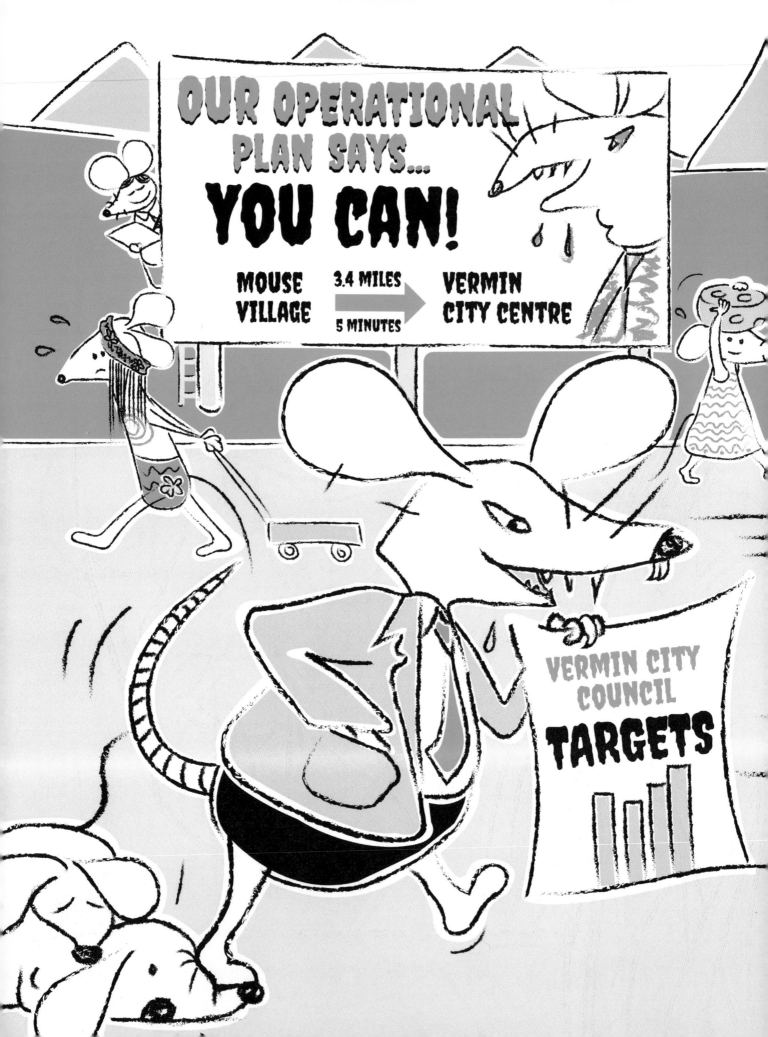

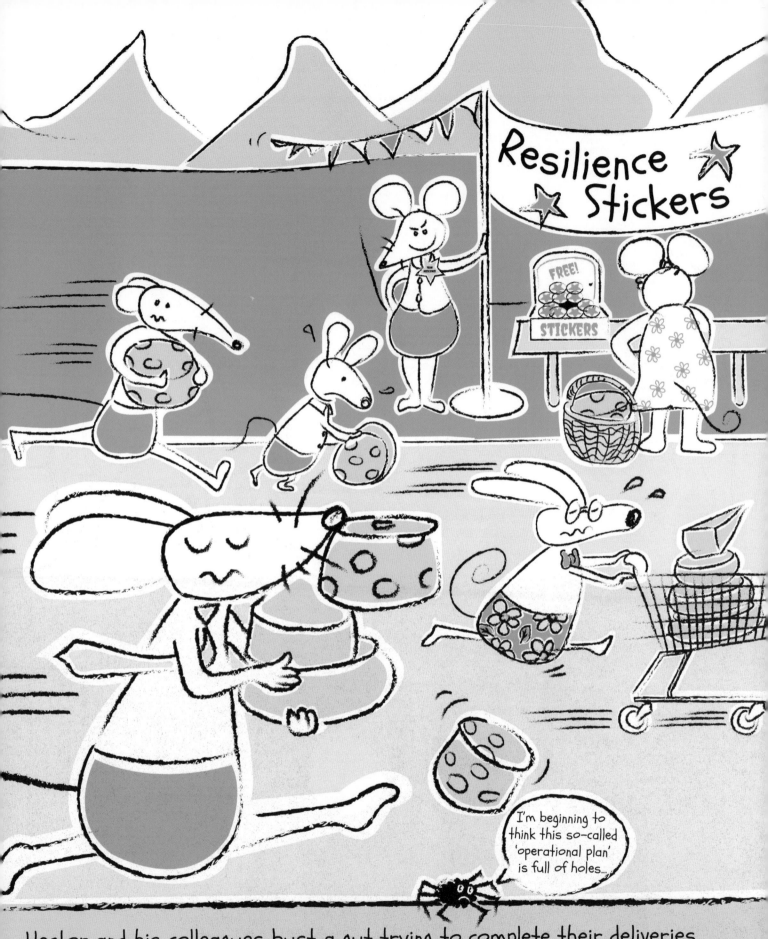

Hector and his colleagues bust a gut trying to complete their deliveries, meet their targets and please their managers. A ready supply of resilience stickers is always available to inspire them on their way!

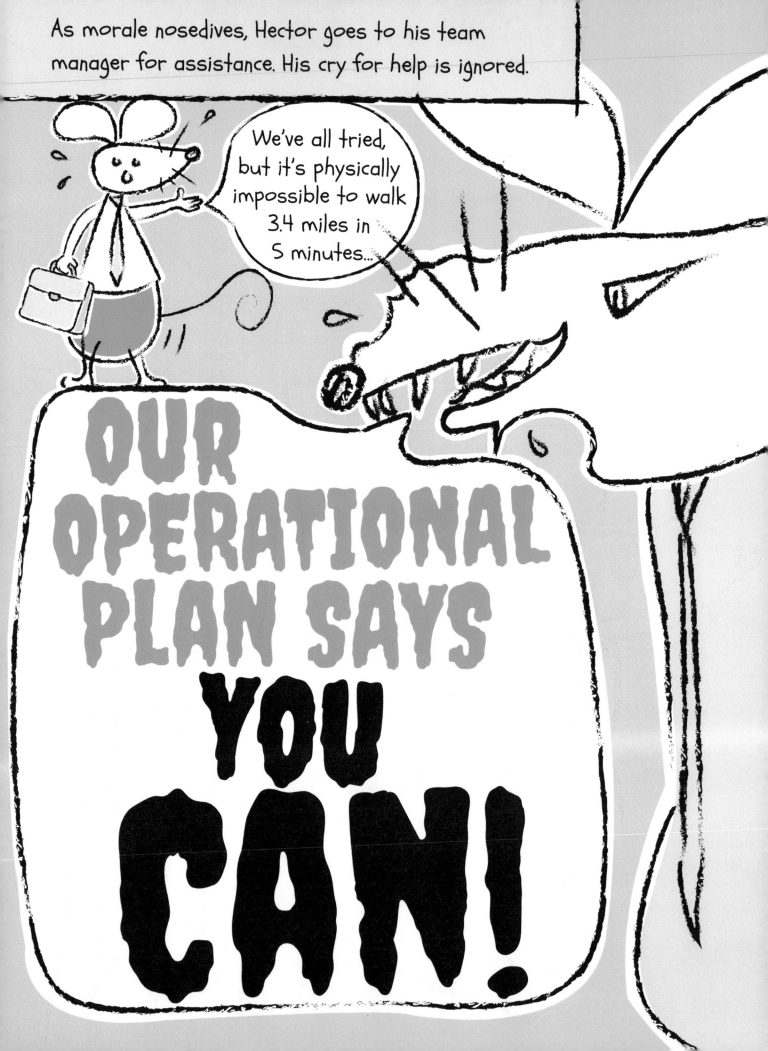

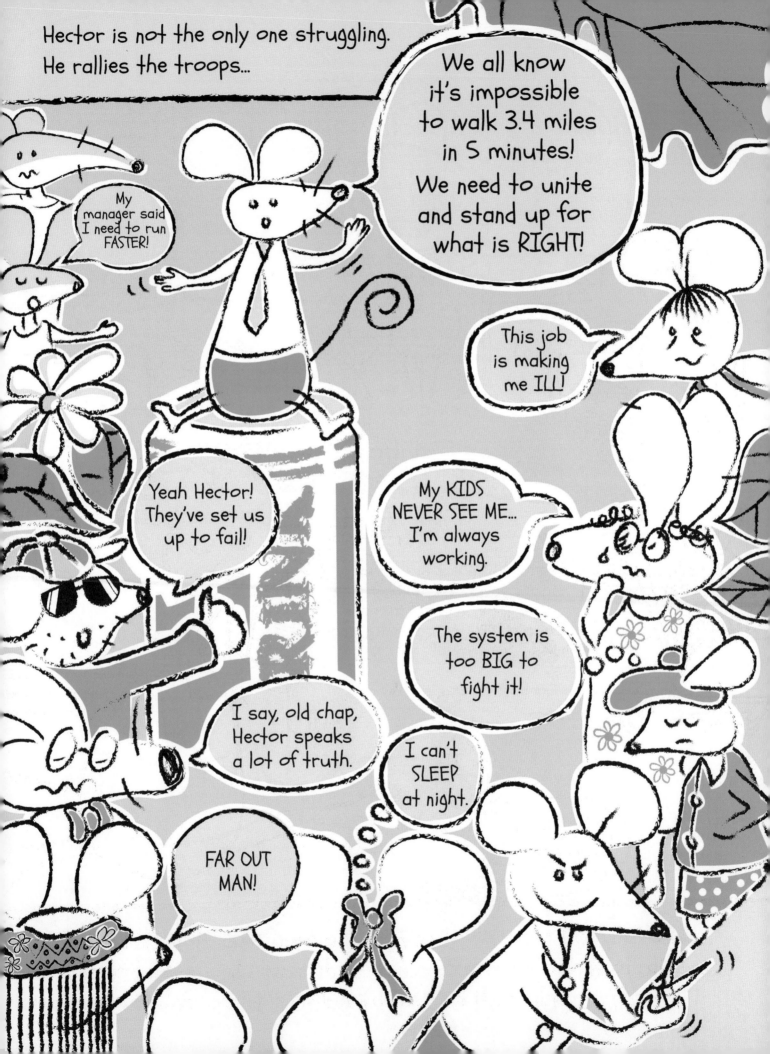

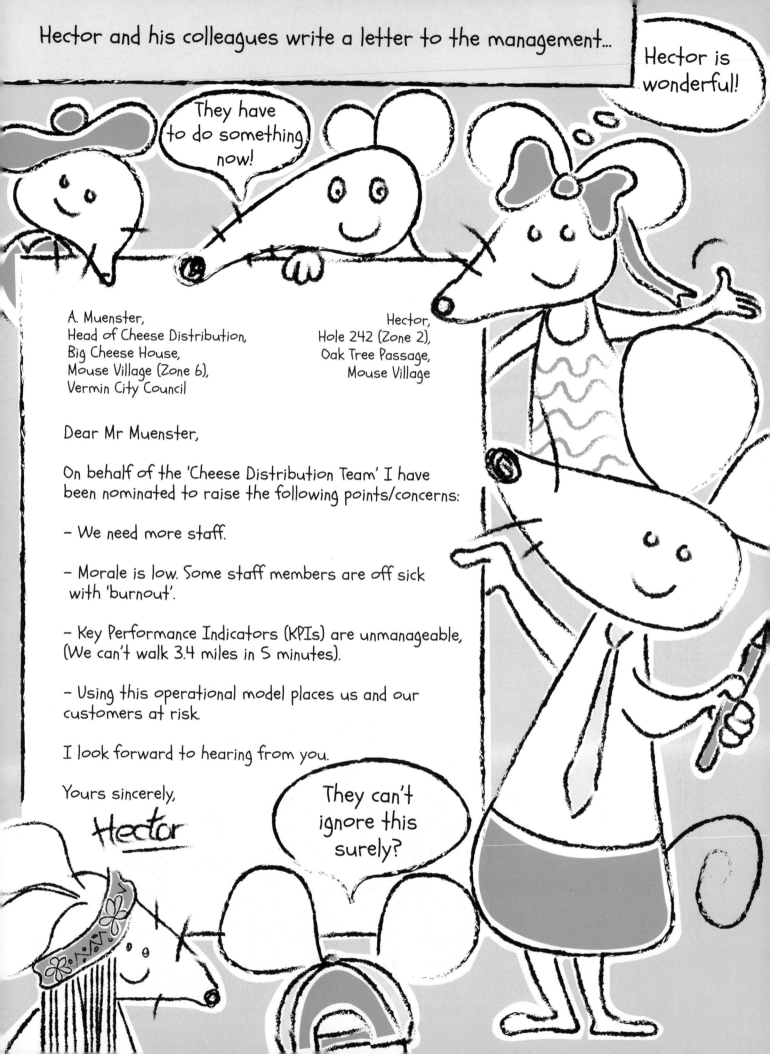

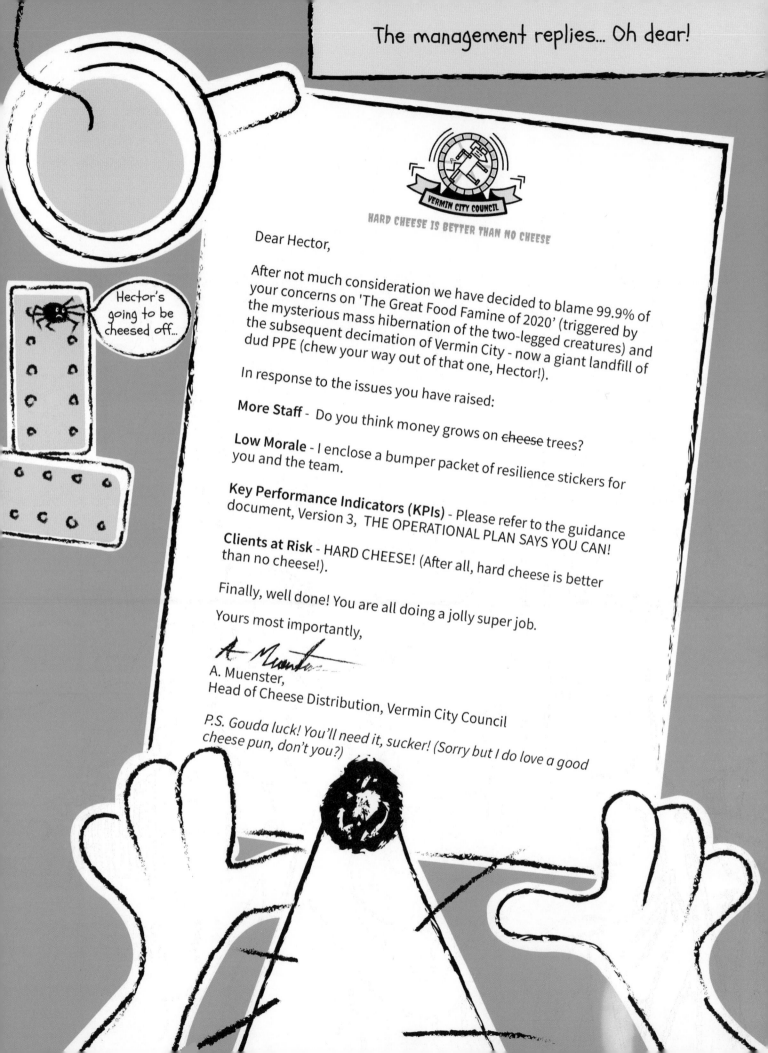

MEETING ROOM
101

PERFORMANCE
MANAGEMENT
SESSIONS

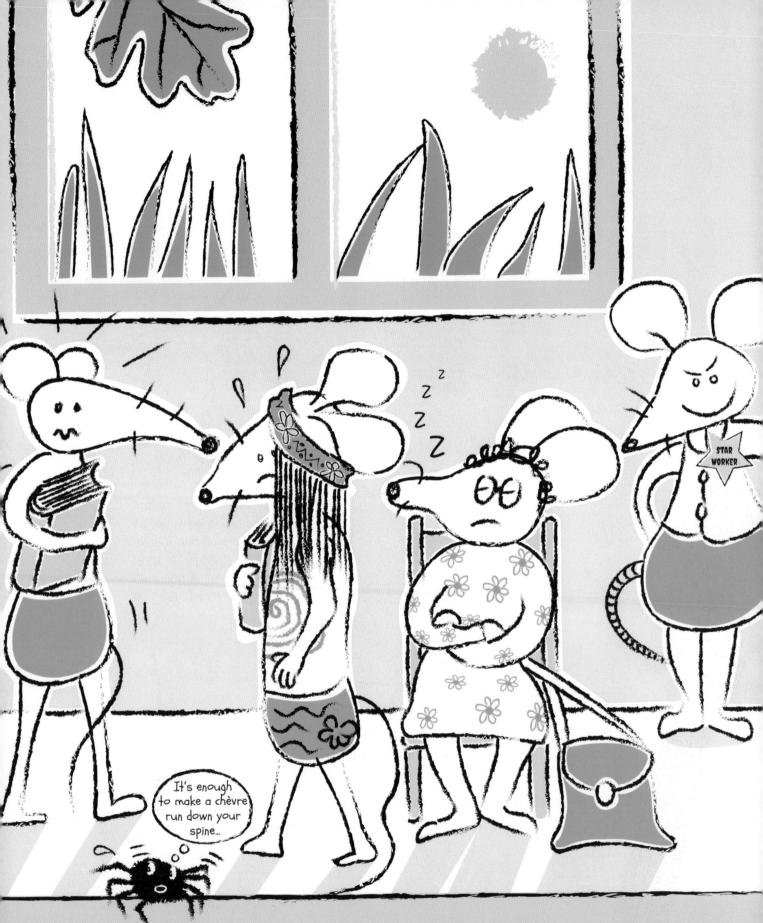

Vermin City Council moves to quash the workers' rebellion by holding Performance Management Sessions – a cunning way to offload responsibility for organisational problems onto the workers.

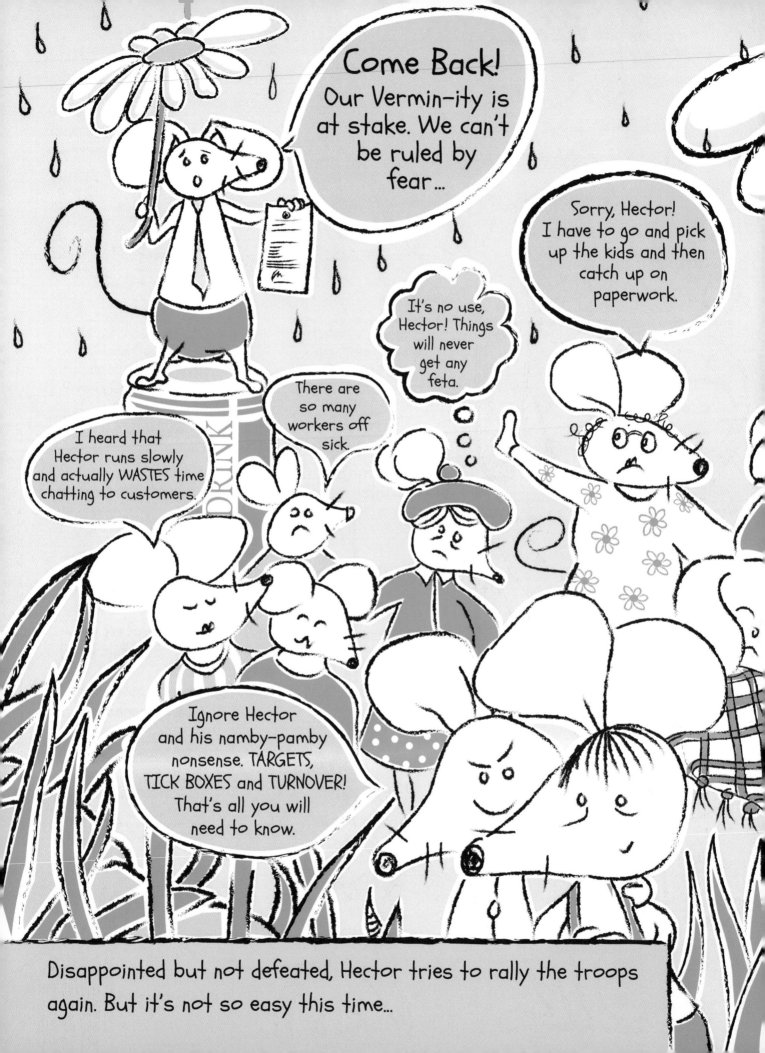

Disappointed but not defeated, Hector tries to rally the troops again. But it's not so easy this time...

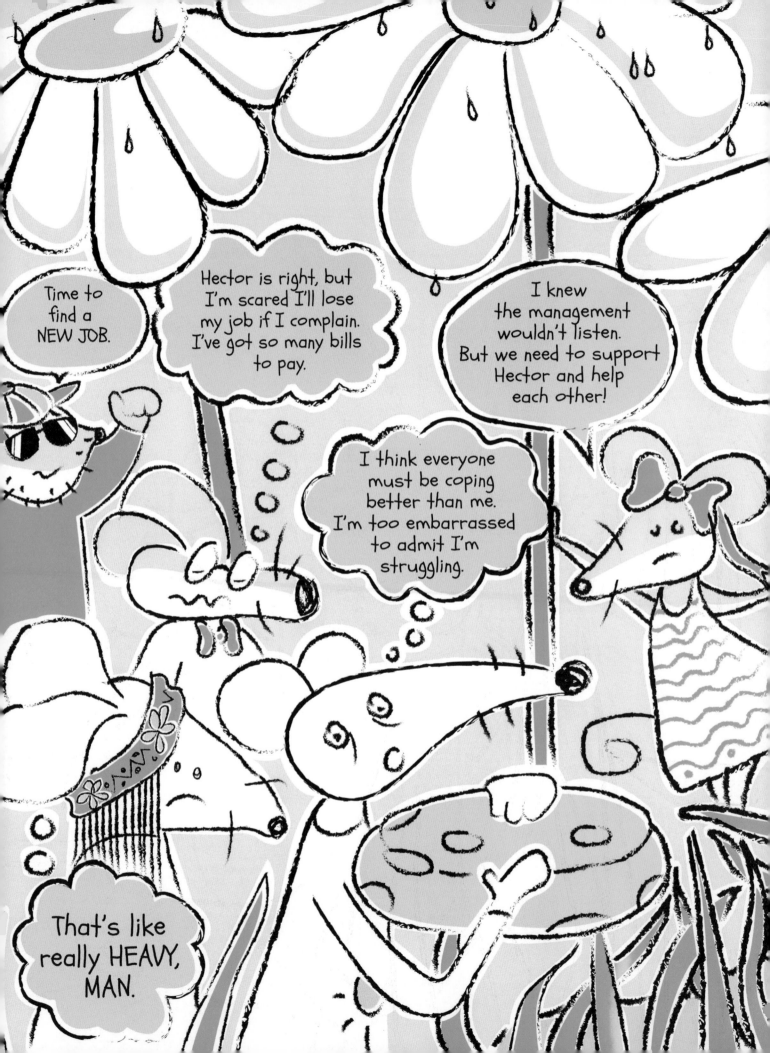

Performance Management Sessions or not, Hector is determined to bring about a change for the better. But not everybody cares about the greater good...

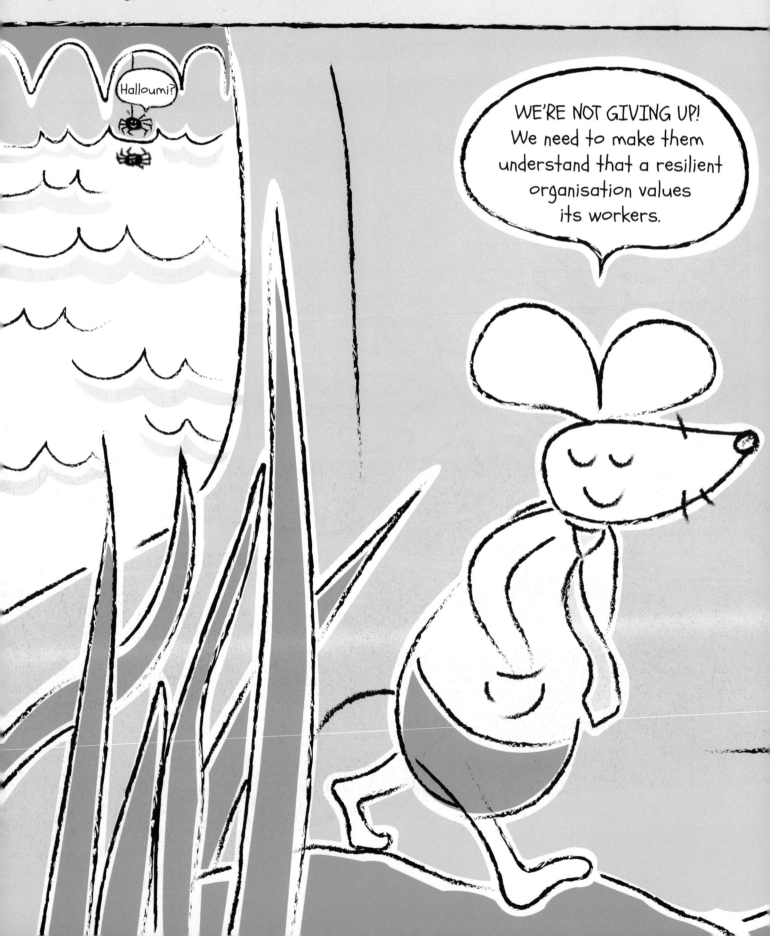

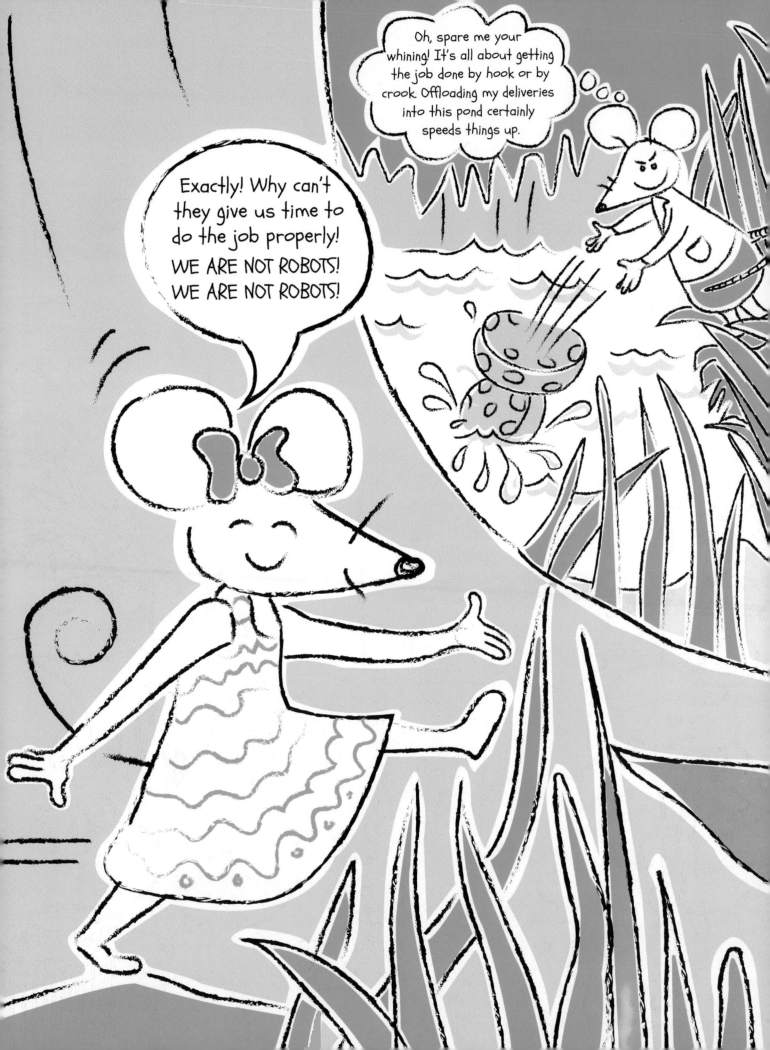

As a loyal employee of Vermin City Council, Hector works 'above and beyond' to support his customers. But the work just keeps on coming ... leaving Hector with no choice but to deliver through the night.

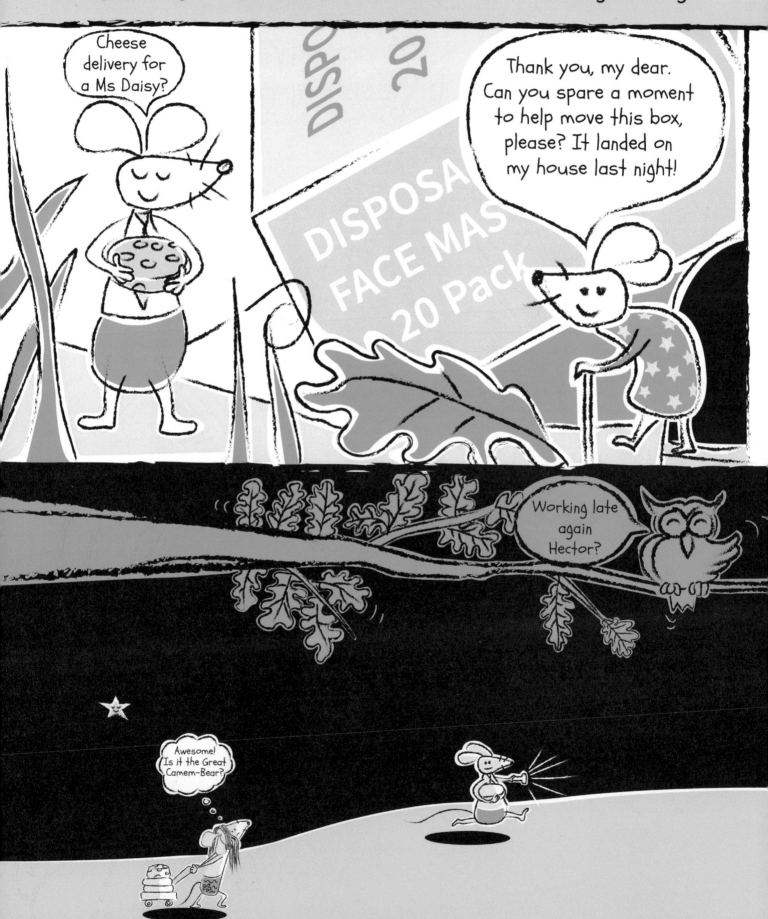

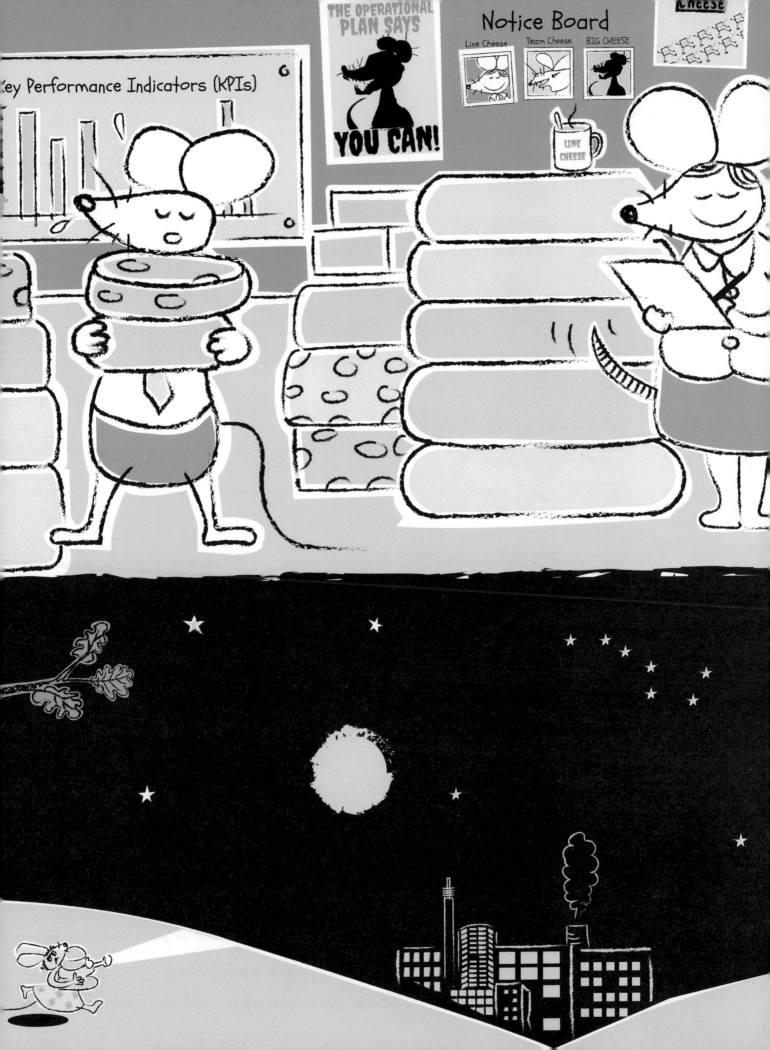

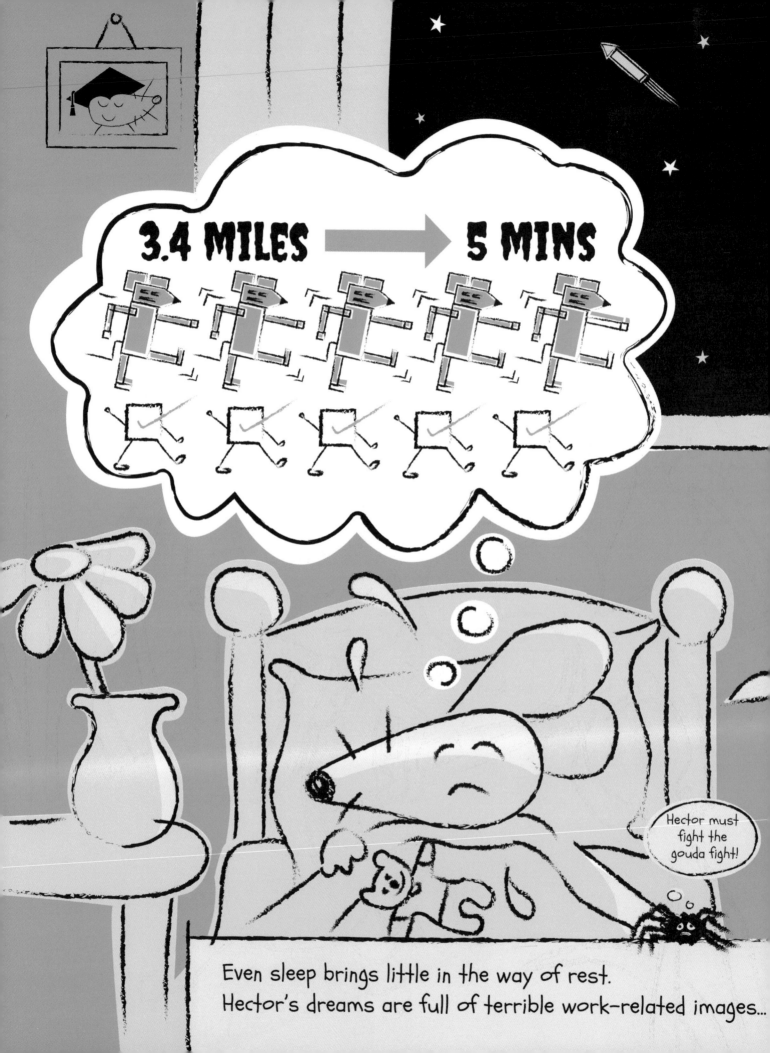

Even sleep brings little in the way of rest.
Hector's dreams are full of terrible work-related images...

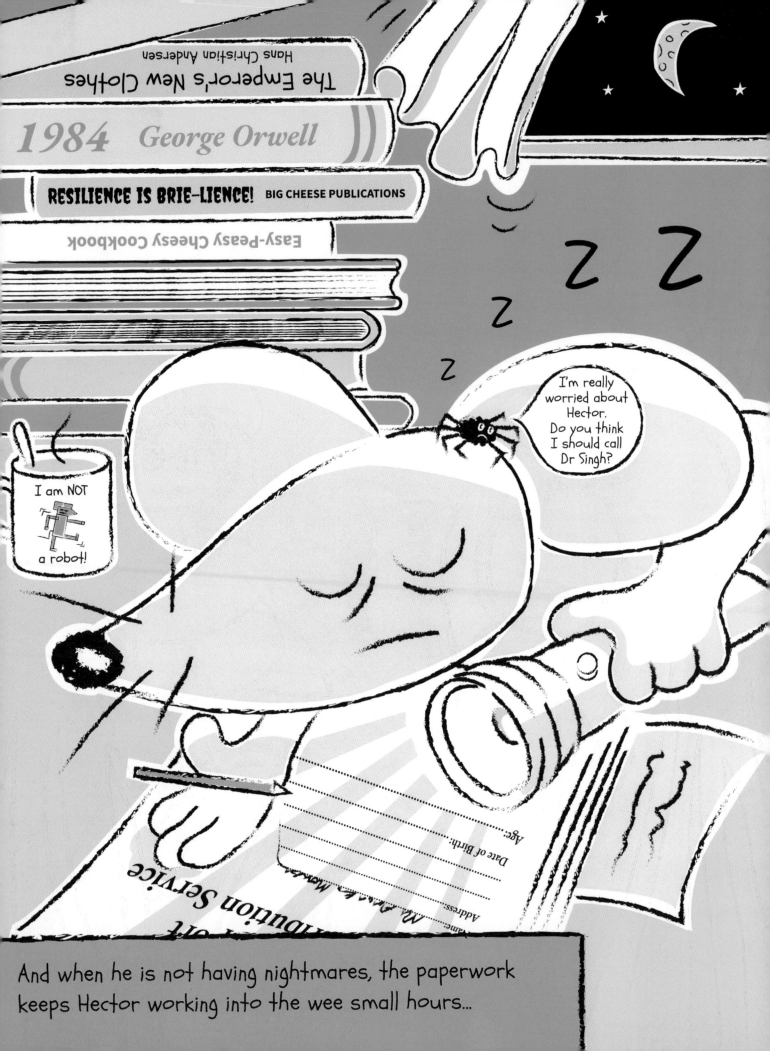

And when he is not having nightmares, the paperwork keeps Hector working into the wee small hours...

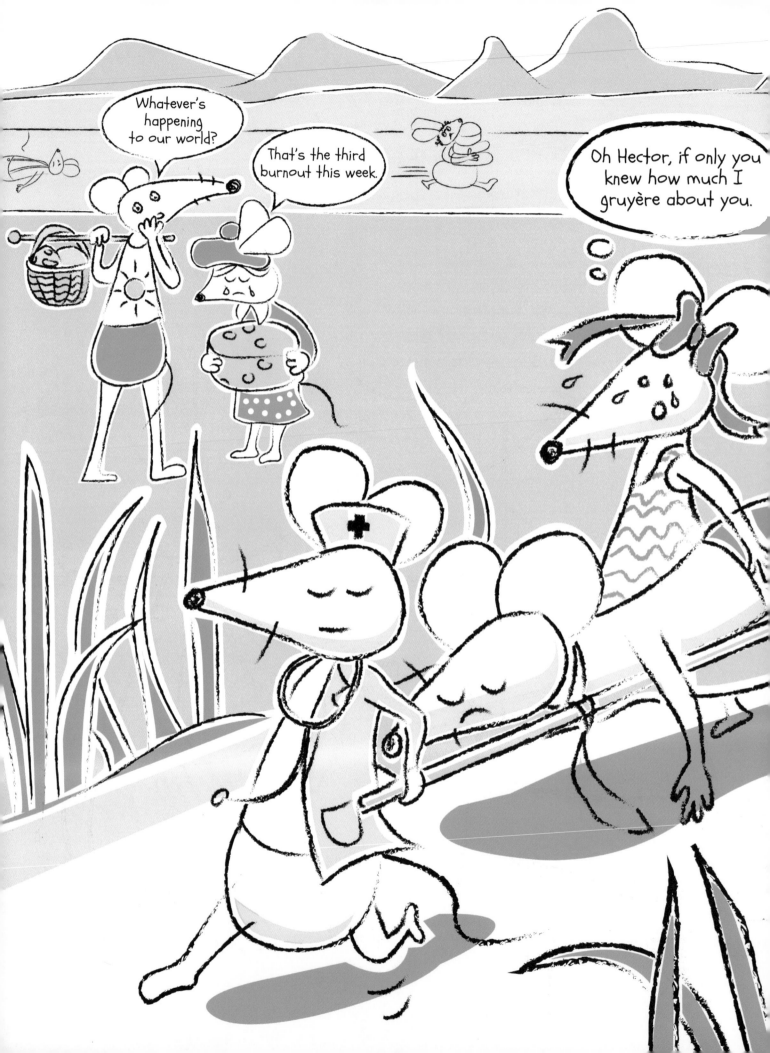

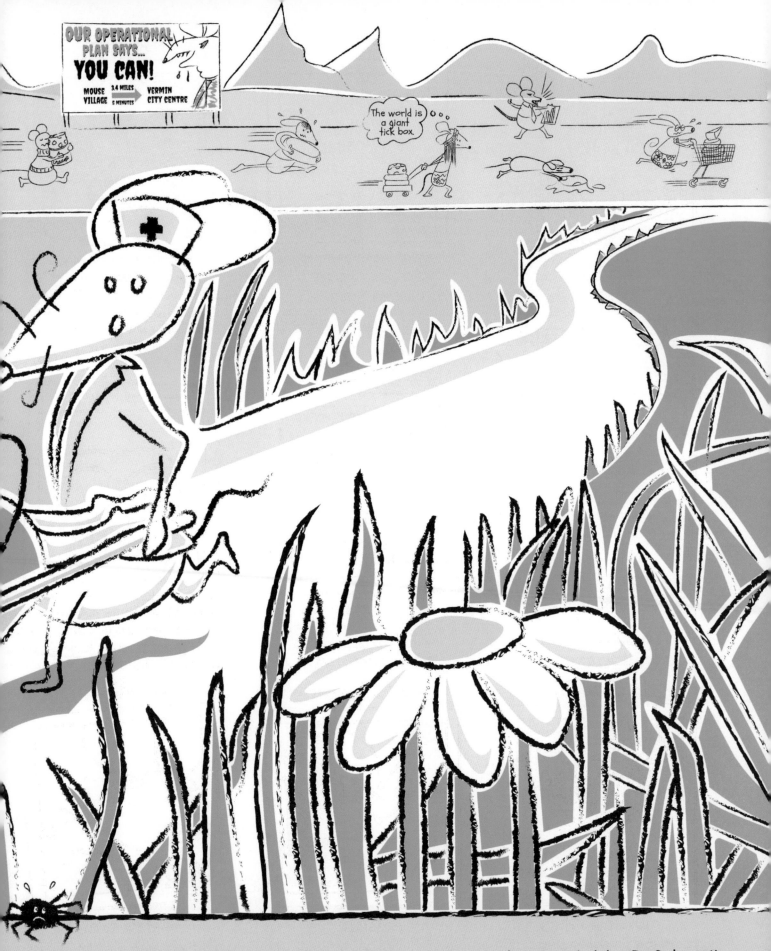

Oh dear! It's happened! Hector finally falls victim to the inevitable 'BURNOUT'! It was only ever going to be a matter of time.

VERMIN CITY COUNCIL

The New Cheese Distribution Team
(plus an owl, a doctor, and a spider ... but minus a Hector)

Hector

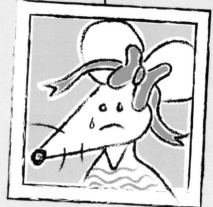

HECTOR IS CURRENTLY UNAVAILABLE. PLEASE CONTACT VERMIN CITY COUNCIL IF YOU HAVE ANY QUERIES.

Sophia

"I hope Hector is going to be okay. He's on sick leave with a diagnosis of burnout. But we're not giving up!"

Alfie

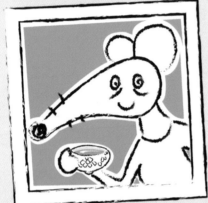

"I'm too ashamed to see Dr Singh, but I've found the best way to cope with this job is a few acorns of fermented nectar after work."

Bal

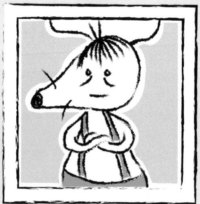

"If I want to survive in this team, I need to be more like Dave. He's so good at ticking boxes."

Azure

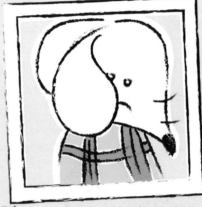

"There is never anybody I can ask for help. There is no time to do the job properly. I have a huge rodent university loan and I feel trapped."

Hebe

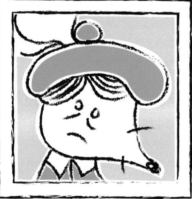

"They told me not to work at night, but then they reprimanded me for not keeping up! So, I must work in my own time, or I'll be blamed if something goes wrong."

Jackson

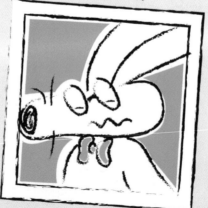

"I have stopped trying to share my ideas as they were 'too ambitious and unrealistic'. I've been getting quite anxious."

Finn

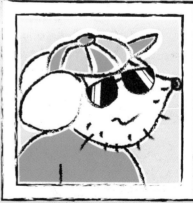

"I'm definitely looking for a new job. But hey, this is 'off the record' so don't be telling the BIG CHEESE!"

Benita

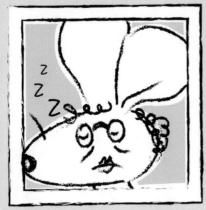

"I'm always working extra hours! I've put on weight, I'm irritable and I feel depressed. I never have time to play with the kids."

Dirty Dave (Promoted!)

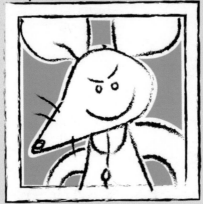

"They quickly recognised I had the right attributes for management. I'll soon be a BIG CHEESE."

Petrichor

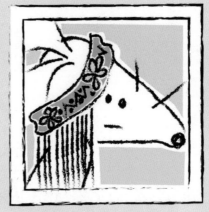

"I'm an old-fashioned worker, not the sort that anyone wants nowadays."

I've donated my space for your story.

Orion

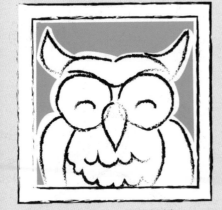

As a wise observer, I would suggest the orgnisational culture of Vermin City Council is undermining the resilience of Hector and his friends."

Dr Singh

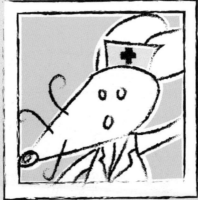

"High cases of worker burnout have been happening for many years, long before 'The Great Food Shortage of 2020'."

(blank frame)

....
....
....

Line Cheese

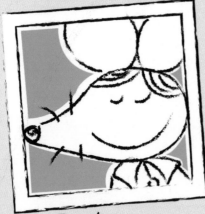

Saccharine

"Our staff members display high levels of resilience and simply bounce back, like rubber balls, in the face of adversity."

Team Cheese

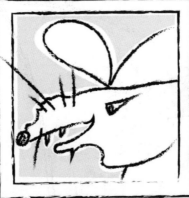

Bernard

"We are all part of a happy and dedicated team, here at Vermin City Council."

BIG CHEESE

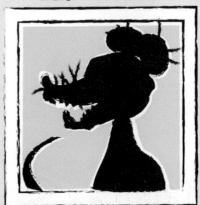

A. Muenster

"This council doesn't run on its provolone, you know! Sorry, but I had to get one in. Now get back to work, pronto!"

The Last Curd

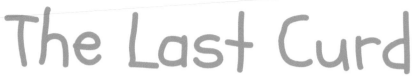

"Burnout is a syndrome conceptualised as resulting from chronic workplace stress that has not been successfully managed." (World Health Organisation, 2019)

In 2021 I experienced occupational burnout, which left me feeling worthless, devalued and isolated. 'Hector' was created as a cathartic release from the stigma of burnout, because I didn't want other hard-working people who experience burnout to struggle alone. Burnout can happen to anyone, at any level, in a multitude of jobs in both the public and private sectors. The World Health Organisation classifies workplace burnout as an occupational phenomenon.

I hope Hector's internal battle resonates with workers. His professional integrity is at stake, as he is expected to compromise his values and conform to a workplace that he believes is flawed and psychologically unsafe. Hector works 'above and beyond' his role. However, he resists his employers' desire for him to take ownership of the failings of Vermin City Council – failings that are perpetuated by a managerialist culture of targets and tick boxes.

Whilst it is tempting to give the story a happy ending (in which Hector sets up an organic cheese shop and discovers his inner self), this would be insulting to those experiencing burnout. In the 'real world', workers have financial responsibilities that tie them to jobs. There is no easy remedy or way out of this cyclical process. Individuals go on sick leave, and it can often be the case that little is done to address the root causes of burnout within their respective organisations. Sometimes the employer may deliver perfunctory 'wellbeing' sessions (a short-term band-aid), enough to tick the respective health & safety boxes. The worker then resumes their work role in the same challenging conditions.

Hector can't offer any quick-fix solutions, but he offers a message of hope: that workers are not alone in their struggles, and collectively we must seek change.

Hmm, who shall I give Hector's workload to?

Psst! Hector told me to tell you, this is definitely not... THE END

cheese

cheese

Printed in Great Britain
by Amazon